The Sleeping Baby Solution

A Complete Training Guide for Baby Sleep and the Perfect Strategies for Sleepless Parents and Stubborn Babies

Rebecca Thomas

Table of Contents

Introduction

Life was going smoothly and everything seemed to be working out just the way you wanted. You had a job, you had a wonderful and supportive spouse, and you had a lovely home that was always warm and inviting. A perfect couple who knew just what the other wanted. You even had a storybook love life to keep things going in the right direction. Finally came the moment where you realized you were about to become a parent. Exciting times, weren't they?

You took your time, bought all the items you might need at the beginning. You bought those fluffy pillows, a cozy baby-sized blanket, caps, mittens, socks, and everything adorable that you could think of. The room was eventually ready to welcome a new member to the family.

Soon enough, the time arrives, you rush to the hospital and prepare for one of the most exciting moments of your life. Your husband is by your side, desperately trying to comfort you. You are going through enormous pain that cannot be explained in words. The doctors come in and say those magic words, "Oh, the baby is ready to come out!"

Lo and behold! After excruciating pushes, rapid breathing and agonizing screams, every sound on earth is halted by your baby's first ever cry. Right there and then, two things happened.

1. You just heard your baby's voice for the first time.

2. You just experienced the most blissful moment of your life.

I am sure most parents or soon-to-be parents knew this already. It is the part that comes next which often puzzles, scares, and even intimidates the unprepared mind.

"Congratulations, you are a parent!" Great... What now?

Parenthood: call it what you may, it is one of the toughest phases in our lives. However, quite a lot of first-time parents tend to focus on the difficulties and how life-altering this phase would be. Let me be the first to tell you that it is okay to be scared. Parenthood is not at all a walk in the park. It takes your entire life to learn how to be a great parent. Growing into your new role as a parent involves constant learning and adapting to changes quickly, as babies grow up fast.

Parenting is both a wonderful aspect of life and a demanding full-time commitment. Babies certainly look cute, adorable, wonderful and all the sweet words you can think of, but it only takes a day for you to realize that you were completely unprepared for some of the major challenges which no one told you about. The biggest challenge, however, is something that is seemingly simple: getting your baby to sleep.

The minute your baby is born, say goodbye to your sleep. I promise you that this is an understatement. If you are a parent and you have no idea how to deal with the constant crying, irregular sleeping patterns, and the continuous hunger of your child, you will not be getting any sleep for quite some time. When you suffer from lack of sleep, you will automatically feel things changing around you. Bad tempers within the house, rough days at work, and coming back home to a baby that is still crying; this is all tough. This is a typical situation parents face when they haven't prepared themselves or equipped themselves with the proper knowledge.

Luckily, we live in a world where information is now available easily. This means that you can search for anything that you may come across during the first few months of parenting, and someone somewhere would have answered it already. The problem arises when you look at the sheer number of responses. It gets extremely hard to distinguish between right and wrong methods, which is why I decided to step in, and hopefully, address the sleep situation once and for all.

Who Should Read This Book?

This book aims to provide facts and information, as well as proven tips and tricks to parents of a child who is under six months of age. If you are a couple who is expecting your child soon, you may have just saved yourself quite a lot of worries. This is not just a parenting guide to teach you how to put your baby to sleep, but also a book that will provide you with some useful tips and suggestions for you to use in order to get some rest.

I have taken every possible measure to ensure that this book is not only informative but also fun to read. A child can get extremely agitated, and there is no way of telling what seems to be wrong with them as the child cannot speak yet.

The book will take you through a journey of learning some of the facts that debunk some myths and old wives' tales that still circle around the internet. We will also look into some essentials which every parent should have, as these can greatly help you along the way.

Furthermore, we will be looking into some of the most common errors parents often end up making, without realizing the potential effects that they would bring. I have made sure to provide you with real-life examples, so that you feel reassurance in knowing that you are not alone. Parents around the globe face most of these issues in exactly the same fashion. It is how they deal with these issues that differ, which is why you are bombarded with thousands of responses found online.

Before We Proceed

All of the information that you will find within this book is meant for educational purposes. Most of these are applicable to every parent. However, there is a rare possibility that a child might suffer from allergies or other complications. If you notice anything unusual such as erratic behavior, or anything that is unexplainable, it is always a good thing to get in touch with a doctor. This book is only to teach you how to put your child to sleep without the use of medicines or herbs. For any health complications, allergies, or other issues, refer to a doctor right away.

I would recommend that you grab a notepad to keep with you as you read. When possible, write down whatever you feel is important or needed. It surely helps to write down important pieces of information so that you can remember what needs to be done when your baby is crying. A quick look and you will know what to do next. With that said, it is time to saddle up, brace yourself, and begin our journey to discover *The Sleeping Baby Solution.*

Chapter 1:
The First Few Signs

For anyone, becoming a parent is one of the greatest feelings on earth. The display of pure love for the child that one feels when the little one holds onto a finger so tightly with their teenie weenie, soft and wrinkled fingers is just out of this world. The minute a parent gets to hold their baby for the first time, a lot goes through their mind. One of these thoughts is a worry; what are parents supposed to do when the baby comes? Well, the baby is here now!

This happened sooner than you thought it would, right? Wrong! You see, as first-time parents, we tend to do a lot of things wrong. The irony is that most of these errors happen after the birth of the child. Don't worry though, I am here to help and walk you through these tough times. Before we do proceed though, I want you to take a deep breath and promise yourself one thing: that you will never give up!

Parenting is extremely hard, I completely understand and can empathize with you. It must be difficult to promise yourself not to give up, given all the sleepless nights you have had to endure. You might be feeling like one of those zombies, straight out of a horror movie, shuffling around with absolutely no sense of direction, purpose, or intent. Some people I know personally quite literally scared me just within a month of being parents. Their faces looked flushed, pale, and quite literally made me feel like the person would jump at me any second to eat me alive.

The problem is the child's unusual sleep habits. Sometimes, a child can sleep for hours while others tend to remain awake with inconsistent sleep patterns. Fatigue can often get in the way of a couple's careers, daily chores, and even their love life. There are many examples that you can find on the internet where couples would report their last intimate encounter being ages ago. When asked for the reason behind such a long gap, most answered, "It's my newborn!"

If you are reading this, there is the likelihood that you too, are suffering from lack of sleep, vigorous mental fatigue, and might even feel like you are about to lose your cool. Stop whatever you are doing, sit down and reassure yourself. Nothing in life is impossible. Besides, that child is just a baby just like you once were. If your parents made it, you can do it too!

Now since we are all set, let us start by observing the obvious. Let us look into some signs that you may have seen and ignored, or may not have seen at all. These signs help you understand what a baby might want. I am not saying these are always the right cases, but I do believe that the science and facts back me up on these tips. On top of that, they have worked for quite a lot of people that I know, and I do not see why these shouldn't work like a charm for you as well!

Know Your Baby's Sleep Pattern and Habits

Newborn babies sleep a lot, and I am not saying nine to 10 hours either. They really do sleep more than you might think. Various sources suggest that newborns sleep around 16 to 17 hours a day.

"What? And I thought I slept a lot." That is exactly what I felt when I first came across this fact.

Considering the staggering number of hours babies tend to sleep, it is only natural to assume that their Rapid Eye

Movement (REM) phase of the sleep cycle differs from that of an adult. You wouldn't be wrong there at all.

We, the adults, have a different sleep cycle. Throughout the cycle, we tend to undergo various phases. Some of these involve changes within our muscular system while some have a profound effect on our brain and neural activities. The REM stage of sleep tends to be only around 25% of the night for adults. This is where we experience vivid dreams, and anyone who is up can tell by noticing the sleeping adult's rapid eye movements. Each cycle lasts between 90 and 120 minutes (How Your Baby's Sleep Cycle Differs From Your Own, n.d.). Babies, well they have a completely unique pattern.

Their sleep cycle is more evenly divided between Non-Rapid Eye Movement (NREM) and REM. Their cycles are shorter as well, as they last only about 90 minutes during the first nine odd months. After that, they are mostly up for a few hours before they go back to sleep again.

Newborn babies tend to sleep a lot because they have just exited their mother's womb. It would take a few weeks before your child starts to be more active, however during that time, there is no need to panic.

There was a couple I came across once in a hospital. They brought their baby in, clearly panicked and worried, stating that their baby wouldn't stay up for more than a few hours at a time before sleeping over and over again. Not so surprisingly enough, it caught my attention. I decided to have a look and saw the nurse doing her thing before breaking out a smile and letting them know it is completely natural for babies to sleep this long. There was nothing wrong with the child, no unusual bumps, no booboos, or anything. Everything was good.

A newborn child needs a bit of time to adjust to their new surroundings. Think of a very, very long flight that you just finished. You traveled thousands of miles into an area with a completely different time zone. What do you think would happen? You would be jet-lagged. It will take some time for you to adjust to the new time zone and until then, you would be sleeping at odd times.

If that sounds fair enough to you, the same goes for the newborn. Just days ago, that child was inside their mother's womb. No light, no sense of who was doing what. Just warmth and coziness is all that the baby felt. Now, the new environment, the harsh light shining brightly across the room, all the noises that the baby never knew existed, all of these factors will cause quite some distraction. Some of these are actually good, while others are a huge 'no' for a baby.

A newborn is quite fragile. Even the slightest movement is enough to wake them up out of a slumber. You might often see your child twitching or jerking, and that is natural. I know that many first-time parents would worryingly rush in and check the baby's vital signs like their heartbeat or whether or not the baby is breathing. Let me tell you that you are only going to make matters worse for yourself. Why? Let's see.

To begin with, a newborn baby has an irregular heartbeat. While we have a normal heartbeat of about 60 beats per minute, their heart beats between 120 to 160 beats per minute. Imagine the horror you would put yourself through when you see your baby twitch a little and you go check their heartbeat and find it beating almost three times as fast as our heartbeats. See what I mean? There was nothing wrong with the baby, to begin with. The baby was snoozing in their cozy little bed perfectly until you decided to jump in and check on them, which ultimately led to your child breaking their slumber.

I haven't even touched on the second part yet. When it comes to breathing, we tend to breathe at a regular pace. We breathe fast when our lungs need more fuel, usually after workouts, sudden scares, and even sexual activity. We breathe slowly when our body is relaxed and at peace, such as when we sleep or even snore. We normally range from around 12 to 20 breaths per minute. Newborns? Well, they are a completely different story.

Newborns breathe around 40 to 60 times in a minute. That is staggeringly high. Even if I want to try out breathing once every second, I would probably pass out halfway through because my lungs wouldn't be getting as much oxygen as I need, yet babies do this exceptionally well. This happens only because their lungs are small, and I mean really small. It wouldn't take much to fill those tiny lungs with air before they are ready to breathe out.

"What's the point of telling me all this?" Well, think about it for a minute. If you had not known these facts, how would you have felt had you gone up to check on your baby and they had an elevated heartbeat and rapid breathing in comparison to your own? I bet you would have called someone or even an ambulance to get things sorted for you and your baby.

It is okay to be afraid of something you have never experienced before. We all learn from our mistakes in one way or another. The good thing is, now you will not panic nor disrupt your child's sleep, and that latter part is the one to focus on. Get that wrong, and everything changes. If I was Janice from Friends, I would be screaming, "Oh my God" and pulling my hair out for not knowing what to do to ease whatever it was that was bothering the child. Once they start crying, it feels like forever before they eventually decide, "You know what, I feel a lot better now" and stop crying. My job is to ensure that you do not go through that same ordeal.

Pick up a notepad, even the one in your cell phone would do. The next few points are essential. Since the baby cannot tell us what the problem is, we need to train ourselves to be Sherlock Holmes and figure out using facts and clues as to what could possibly be causing our dear child to cry so loud. We will be creating a checklist, which you can use multiple times. Use it to do some quick routine checks to eliminate doubts and find the actual cause. Focus on the ones you answer 'no' to as those could possibly be the culprit behind their crying.

1. Has the baby taken a nap? Believe it or not, most of the time a child cries when their body feels tired. They just want to go to sleep. If only we could do that at times, too. Naps are important, and it is mostly through naps that babies complete their 16 to 17 hours of sleep per day. If it has been more than two hours since the baby last slept, and the baby has taken a dose of milk, priority one is to put the baby to rest.

2. Is the baby feeling comfortable? There is a big difference between what we believe is comfortable and what is actually comfortable for a baby. If a baby is wearing tight clothing, perhaps loosen them up a bit. A good habit would be to stick to soft and comfortable clothing. Care must be taken though as some materials which may seem comfortable might activate allergies. If you spot redness anywhere on the body, stop using that fabric right away. If the clothing seems comfortable and the baby is still crying, move on to the next points.

3. Is their diaper clean? Babies do not like being in dirty diapers for long. Besides, it is always recommended that you change their diaper as soon as it is dirty. Leaving

your baby in dirty diapers for long can expose them to rashes. Rashes can increase the frustration and the agony that the child might go through.

4. If their diaper is clean, check for rashes just in case. If you see rashes around the buttocks, use the appropriate ointment, or consult a doctor. This is a fairly common problem and almost every child develops rashes at some point in time. Once again, there is nothing to be alarmed about but you can certainly avoid frequent rashes by keeping your baby clean.

5. Check if your baby is too hot or too cold. Babies have super sensitive skin, resulting in them getting too cold or growing too warm rather quickly. Touch their arms, ears, nose, and forehead to determine if they are feeling uncomfortable due to temperature. Your baby may have a fever or might be feeling too cold.

This checklist would normally narrow the cause down and you should be able to find the source that is causing your dear child to stay up and cry. However, there are some other things you can do to ease the baby's crying.

Sometimes, when infants are still breastfed, it is normal that some of the milk may have rolled off their cheek. The milk can make your baby feel wet around their neck area and which can cause your baby to feel agitated. Use a clean cloth to wipe any spills and soon enough, your baby should be cooing those beautiful sounds before they fall asleep.

It is also advisable to ensure that after every feed, you should make sure that your baby burps. I am sure you already know this, but what happens if you do not make them burp immediately after a feed?

Normally, your baby burps to signal that they have digested the milk or feed. There are some circumstances where they may not burp, and that is normal at times as well. However, it does mean that pretty soon your baby will have some gas build-up in their tummy. If their tummy hurts due to gas, the baby will cry, leaving you clueless because there would be no visible sign of anything being wrong. If this happens, gently rub their belly until the baby either burps or farts. Yes, babies fart too, but that's not the point.

To massage, lay your baby down on their back and start gently rubbing their tummy in a clockwise motion. This is to ease the trapped gas to move in the right direction. Gradually, pull your hands down the curve of their belly. This further helps any trapped gas to move ahead and it should ease the baby's tummy almost immediately. You can repeat these motions several times until the baby is no longer crying.

Once all is done, the baby should start rubbing their eyes, indicating the need to sleep or nap. Presto! You just made your baby sleepy. Well done!

No! We're Not Done Yet!

To ensure your baby sleeps peacefully, there are a few things to consider. Get these right and your baby would be fast asleep in no time. Ready then? Let's go.

Swaddle

Oh, how I love saying that word. For those who may not know what swaddle is, it is nothing too complicated. It is just a way to wrap your baby up nice and tight, giving them the feeling of warmth and coziness that they experienced in the womb.

By wrapping up a baby correctly, it can make them calm and promote sleep (American Academy of Pediatrics). So how do you swaddle a baby then? Follow these simple steps and you should be able to swaddle your baby up nicely.

1. Spread the blanket out on a flat surface, and fold one corner.

2. Lay the baby on top of the blanket, face-up, with their head just above the folded corner.

3. First, straighten the baby's left arm and wrap the left corner of the blanket over the body. Tuck it in right between the right arm and the right side of the body.

4. Now, tuck the right arm down, fold the right corner of the blanket over the body, and right under the left side.

5. You can either twist or fold the bottom side of the blanket. However, this part needs to be done loosely. Do not tighten the bottom side. Tuck it under one side of the baby.

6. Make sure that the blanket isn't too tight and that the hip region can move should the baby want to move a bit. A rule of thumb would be to have at least two or three fingers fitted between the swaddle and the baby's chest.

Swaddling your baby is effective and is more than just an ancient technique to put babies to sleep. The American Academy of Pediatrics also vouch for this technique and consider it to be effective in promoting sleep for infants.

Once your baby starts to show signs of trying to roll over, that is the point where you must stop swaddling your baby. This is generally around two to three months of age. By now, your baby would have already reduced their hours of sleep and developed a more predictable sleeping pattern. Don't get me wrong though, they will still sleep more than we do, but soon they will find the right rhythm.

Swaddling your baby does come with some risks. These cases are rarely observed but when they do, it is because one may have swaddled the baby incorrectly. There are some safe sleep recommendations for parents who wish to swaddle their babies. Follow these and hopefully, you should never have to worry about any of the potential risks.

- Always ensure that you place your baby on their back to sleep. While doing so, observe to see if your baby is trying to roll. If so, you can no longer safely swaddle your baby.

- Keep an eye out for any loose blankets within the baby's crib. Loose blankets can easily come undone and could potentially fall on the child's face, thus increasing the risk of suffocation.

- The AAP states that specialized mattresses, wedges, sleep surfaces, and all the other fancy and rather expensive baby care products have failed to show any signs of reducing the risk of Sudden Infant Death Syndrome. That means that there is no reason to spend such a large amount of money on things that aren't proven to reduce the risk of SIDS.

- The baby is always, and I mean always, the safest within the crib. Your bed is not safe for such a small child yet, even when swaddled.

- When swaddling, it is possible that your child may feel hot. Keep an eye out for signs of damp hair, sweat, flushed cheeks, or even rapid breathing. If you spot any of these signs of overheating, remove their blankets and any excess clothing items to normalize the baby's body temperature.

- Your baby should always sleep in a smoke-free area. No excuses there.

There are things that may seem promising at first but may not work right away. Patience is the key here. It takes quite a lot of it as well. Do not get yourself caught up in the "let's try this as well" mindset just yet. If plan 'A' fails, try again. You will need to persevere and struggle a little because everything is new for your baby. The baby will take some time to adjust to their surroundings, those strange new feelings, light conditions, and noises. Once the baby is settled, the results will be far more rewarding.

Now then, we went through some first signs, made a small checklist, and even learned what swaddling is. Give yourself a pat on the back for making it this far in the book for the sake of your child. The ultimate reward of getting some well-earned rest is now one step closer. We aren't there yet, but soon we will be.

You will be able to watch your darling little one sleep peacefully, and in the process, you will have a peaceful sleep after such a long time yourself. Keep that motivation up high and I assure you, we will make it through just fine.

Chapter 2:
Baby - Most Effective Communicator

Communication is the key to our success. Whether on a personal level or in a professional setting, effective communication is vital and stands between you and your success. Get your message clearly across the board and you would walk out with a massive smile on your face stretching from east to west. Get it wrong, and of course, the results would be rather disappointing.

In our daily lives, we communicate almost every single minute of the day. We know what we want, we know how to tell someone what we want, and we know the ways to tell someone how we are feeling. Effective communication is straightforward and honest. But what about the new member of the family? How can an infant who can barely even say goo-goo-ga-ga communicate with us? How can a baby tell us what they want, need, or desire? The answer is exactly what you might be thinking; they cry!

While the professionals of the world try and make a fortune off of being effective communicators, no one is better at communicating than an infant. Every cry that comes out of that tiny little mouth is pure, honest, and free of any influences. It is a direct cry to demand something.

A baby knows only one way to communicate and it comes to them naturally: making noises. These noises can be a giggle, a cry, or even those funny sounds that they make when they are feeling playful and jolly.

A child's mind is pure and honest. It is not surrounded by questions which we often end up with when making a decision. We constantly ask ourselves 'if' it would be okay to ask for a leave from the boss, 'if' it would be okay to ask for some snacks from a friend. These 'ifs' are non-existent, which is why a baby simply communicates without a second thought. The problem is, the baby may be an effective communicator, but we are not experts and we can clearly not understand what they want from their limited sound bank of noises and cries. Once again, persevere and you might just start seeing a pattern. Besides, you have this book, right?

A Noise Can Mean Many Things

If your child is a few days old, they may not do anything except try to yawn, cry, throw up a little, drink, and sleep. However, if your child is a month or two old, there is a good chance that they have started to make some new noises. They may sound like small and adorable efforts of a child trying to scream in excitement, tiny little giggles, or even surprisingly loud cries. In either case, every noise your child makes means something.

Babies are known to make a variety of noises. These range from baby babbles to grunts and giggles, not to forget the cries. Surprisingly, most of the time, these babies are fascinated by the new world that they are experiencing every day. You may have noticed how the baby continues to look around the room, look at people, and then look back at you. They are familiarizing themselves at this stage. They may not know who you are right away, but the minute you hold them, there exists this magical bond that immediately connects the baby to you, the parent.

During these times of exploration, the baby can often be disturbed by quite a few things. These can include the bright lights, the sudden increase in noise level, or even a common housefly landing on top of their forehead. Everything is new, and the only few ways a baby can respond to their surroundings are sound-based. It is through these sounds that parents can learn what seems to fascinate the child and what seems to do the opposite. You may wish to start paying attention to your baby's stage and find out what may seem to be working. If your child can move about a little, you may wish to let them hold a toy and see how they react to it. Try and listen to their change in tone and the noises that they use to show excitement or happiness. A baby may often use these sounds to indicate that they feel happy or that they want their toys.

Since we are talking about sounds, it would be extremely useful if you were to somehow learn of a few sounds which kids normally make. I am not talking about the laughter or the cry here, I mean actual sounds. We normally disregard these as nothing but gibberish, but thorough research and study have been conducted on these sounds to prove otherwise.

Priscilla Dunstan, the Australian Opera singer who is famously known for the creation of Dunstan Baby Language, observed and studied babies from around the world for eight whole years before coming to a conclusion. Her conclusion showed that every baby, regardless of race, color, cultural background, and gender, makes one of the following five sounds just before they are about to cry. That sound is a key indicator in understanding what the baby wants. These sounds are:

- **Neh -** To denote that the child is hungry

- **Eh -** When the child needs to burp

- **Eairh -** When the child wishes to pass gas

- **Heh -** To show some form of discomfort, such as being wet, hot or cold

- **Owh** - When the baby is sleepy

Now, the problem is that these noises are pretty hard to comprehend the first few times. All the sounds feel exactly like each other, differentiating these can be rather difficult. Fortunately, there are other ways as well. Let us look at these one more time, but this time with their alternative actions included.

- The **'Neh'** sound is made by a baby to let you know that it is time for them to feed. If you may have missed it, do not worry. The alternative is quite easy and apparent. You may see a baby trying to gnaw or even suck on their hand. If you are a mother, the baby may try to reach for your breast, or somewhere in that general area. These are significant signs that indicate that the baby is hungry. I picked up one more way to find out if the child is feeling hungry. Tap your index finger just above the upper lip a few times gently. If your baby tries to chase it and opens her mouth, voila! The baby is hungry!

- The **'Eh'** sound is very similar to the previous one. If you miss this one as well, I wouldn't be surprised. Everybody tends to miss these noise cues at first. This sound isn't exactly a voluntary act though. This is more of a distress signal that is caused by a bubble of air trapped within the baby's chest. The baby does the 'Eh' sound in an attempt to somehow release this uncomfortable bubble of air. The alternative, however, is quite visible and easily understood. The baby would show a pained facial expression, shaking their arms, kicking their feet, squirming, or even moving hips. If you try and offer the other breast or some bottled milk, they may turn it away which is a clear indicator that something is bothering them from the inside. Burp your baby as needed, and they should be all set once again.

- The '**Eairh**' sound is more of a reflex that passes information about a potentially upset tummy. The problem with this one is that the sound, if you miss it, is followed by loud, intense, and rhythmic crying. The baby will cry out quite loud and that alone should be an indicator that the baby has an upset tummy. They may even raise their legs to their tummies or arch their backs or just be fidgety in general. The baby will stop crying as soon as the gas is passed. Use the clockwise massaging technique we learned in the first chapter and all the tummy aches should go away.

- The '**Heh**' sound is also a reflex sound. This sound generally shows that the baby is not exactly comfortable. This could be due to a few reasons such as a full diaper or feeling cold. This sound is probably the easiest to miss as most of the sounds a baby would make resemble this one. The alternative isn't exactly easy to spot either. They will cry mildly and intermittently. If you know your child's cry and you can spot the difference between the previous one and this one, you would know right away that it is not a tummy ache but possibly something much smaller and easier to fix. The crying will only intensify if you ignore their calls so be sure to soothe the baby right away.

- The '**Owh**' sound. Guess what? It is yet another reflex sound. It sounds quite similar to a yawn and is quite easy to pick out. Alternatively, a baby may start rubbing their eyes, or they may cry slow and low. However, ignore the call and the cry can pick up intensity. If your baby is tired and exhausted, the cry would be intense right from the start. It is quite easy to misinterpret as well. You might start massaging their belly when they really need to sleep. The key to catch the difference is to pick up the sound and the signs before they start to cry.

These five sounds and the alternative actions should provide you with enough to go on. Use these to tackle most situations and get your baby to sleep easily. Some of the most common issues when putting a baby to sleep include not knowing what your baby might want at that point in time. If your baby is hungry, and you are trying to put them to sleep instead, it is all going to end up in a big disaster.

These sounds are hard to catch, but as I mentioned earlier, you do everything but quit. It takes a bit of practice but I assure you, soon you will not be guessing because you will know every sound your baby makes and determine what they want. The quicker you tend to your baby's needs, the quicker the baby can go to sleep.

Your Child's Responses to Sounds

Apart from the noises a baby makes, there are other noises that go on in the background. These play a huge role in every baby's life.

Sounds that are gentle, pleasing, and designed for kids are generally the ones that promote your child to either be excited or feel cozy and sleepy. Other sounds, like that of a blender or a car alarm, or even something heavy falling down can bring the opposite results. These sounds can easily startle a child even if they are fast asleep. Children have one of the most active hearing abilities on earth. They are able to pick up and respond to the smallest of sounds quickly and easily. Even if they are asleep, they can hear most noises with no problems at all. This then leaves parents with their work cut out for them.

To put the baby to sleep, one thing is certain; you will quite literally need to remove all sources of distraction. It is a very common sight to come across a baby that is sleeping peacefully and one of the toys in their room falls over somehow. The baby would be startled and quite literally twitch and shake briefly but violently. First-time parents can often find themselves scared to see just how badly a child reacts to sounds during their sleep. It is normal, but that does not mean that you stop worrying about it. These sudden changes and body movements can often lead to sprains, pulled muscles, and other issues. Try your best to keep your baby in the most comfortable, quiet, and peaceful place possible to ensure they get to sleep well.

Every baby pays close attention to the sounds that they hear around them. Surprisingly, their hearing begins even before their birth. While they can hear the sounds of the world outside the womb, being in the outside world and listening to these sounds is a completely different experience.

Babies respond well to familiar voices such as those of their parents and siblings. Any loud or unexpected noises will startle your child and they may respond with a sudden movement. Whenever you see that your baby is startled, it is a good idea to calm them down so that they feel safe and protected.

A baby that is around two months old will start going quiet whenever they come across a familiar sound. This is natural as they will then try to listen and respond to these sounds. Most of the time, they may start using vowel sounds like, "oh." It is a good indicator that your baby's hearing ability is good if they respond to these sounds and say something, or at least try to chase the sound by looking around for the source. If your baby looks away or fails to respond a few times, have your baby's hearing examined by a doctor.

While it is rare, it is still a possibility that a child may not be able to hear the sounds correctly, especially if the sounds are loud which would otherwise startle any other baby. Having an expert observe the child can lead to some clues and hopefully resolve the issue early on.

When your baby grows to around four months of age, they are now able to chase the source of noises more easily. At this stage, the baby has developed some more muscles, allowing them more mobility and movement. By the sixth month, they will start imitating these sounds. At this stage, a baby will also stop getting startled as frequently as they once did a few months ago. The involuntary reflex of throwing their arms and legs will eventually cease and they would rather resort to crying.

The sense of hearing can be quite helpful for parents to use in order to promote sleep and calmness. There are many crib toys and music-based items which further help babies feel sleepy. They are also a good source if you want to calm the baby when he or she is crying for seemingly no reason. It is normal for babies to be stubborn at times, and toys can make life a lot easier.

The responses that your child shows to specific sounds can often come in handy. Use the ones that clearly comfort them and avoid the ones which may startle them during their sleep. Do this right, and you should have no problem putting your baby to sleep and perhaps take some time for your partner as well. Trust me, the love life takes a hit and it is often quite hard to find the right time where partners can engage in some intimacy when babies are up and crying.

Early childhood is where parents train themselves by adjusting their activities according to the needs of the child. Once the child starts walking and talking, things can get a lot easier and you can then teach your child. At this point in time, your infant does not learn much but only responds in certain ways. Contrary to popular belief, toys are not going to teach your kids much either. It is only when they start speaking and communicating a bit that they begin their learning phase.

All the above that I mentioned is good, but how can you tell if your baby is willing to play or somehow communicate with you? Easy! Babies quickly learn the ability to flex their muscles and muster a little smile. Additionally, they wiggle their hands, fingers, and toes to show excitement. This may be triggered by some source of noise such as one of those overhead hanging crib toys or a parent trying to make funny faces. However, when you feel the child is drowsy, stop making such noises which might reignite curiosity within the child. This may prevent them from sleeping and pretty soon, they will feel irritated and cranky. That is an indication that a child's body is tired and exhausted.

Turn off all the sources of noise such as music from toys, and ask others to stay quiet until the baby is well asleep. Do not put your baby in their crib right away. Ensure that the baby is fast asleep and then lower them into the crib, gently. Any sudden move or noise will wake them up and that may lead to another long session of the baby crying and you trying to calm them down.

To further help you with this, you can follow this list which shares what kind of noises startle or excite babies at a specific age. You can add these to your notepad and use it, later on, to help you avoid these sounds when the baby is sleeping or feeling drowsy:

- **After birth (Newborn)** - Simple loud noises such as a hand clap or perhaps the 'thud' sound of a door slamming shut. These are enough to cause your baby to open their eyes widely and perhaps even start to cry.

- **One month old** - The baby at this age will notice any sudden and prolonged noises. These may include routine noises like turning the vacuum cleaner on. The baby will pause and try to focus on the noise.

- **Four months old** - The baby at this age will show signs of excitement upon hearing familiar sounds. They may even turn their heads around to find the source. They may take a little bit of time to find the source, but once they do, their excitement will be off the charts.

- **Nine months old and above** - Listens attentively and seeks out the source themselves almost instantly. They will respond to their names and may use a word or two depending on their interest.

Sounds play an important role for newborns and babies up to a year old. Sounds are essentially the first of many things that will draw their attention, provoke a response, and allow the child to somehow interact accordingly. Use the appropriate sounds to further add to the situation. If a child is fresh and full of energy, use playful sounds, or use baby talk to get their attention and let them know that it is playtime. To put them to bed, use sounds or musical melodies which promote their sleep. Over time, a child will grow accustomed to these sounds and will go to sleep a bit quicker.

There you have it, you now know almost every concept that makes a baby one of the most effective communicators on the planet. They are honest in expressing their emotions. On top of that, you also learned how they respond and communicate, in their own way, when faced with various sounds. Their little words may seem indistinguishable at first, but each holds a different meaning.

Involve your partner and try to practice picking up these tiny details as these will allow you to understand the baby better and provide the baby with exactly what they need when they need it. The sooner that happens, the sooner you can enjoy your rest.

In the next chapter, I will be focusing on a few errors and myths which many have come to believe to be true. Some of these may be effective but some are highly unlikely to work. Why should we look into these, I hear you ask? Simple! You will save a lot of your time and energy by avoiding things that are only going to lead you into a world of issues, leaving you with only the methods and techniques which genuinely work. And that means the little one will not have to stay up and wait for you to figure out what needs to be done longer than needed.

Chapter 3:
You Probably Shouldn't Do That

We live in a world that is virtually encompassed with data flowing in every direction you can see. Our parents had no way of accessing such a large database, leaving them with all the guesswork and many myths to debunk before finding out what works for a baby and what doesn't.

Today, fortunately, we are just a stroke of a button away from some of the finest, most detailed information you can ask for. The internet is truly our friend, and an incredible way of finding out whatever it may be that is bothering you... or is it?

Imagine going to a library to search for a book that could help you understand what is keeping your baby up at night, and for a second, let's pretend that doctors aren't available anywhere near us. You walk into a library and you are stunned to find the sheer size of the shelves, stretching on for miles after miles, with no end in sight. To make matters worse, every book in this massive library is about the same thing you are seeking. What do you think would happen?

For starters, you would be left completely puzzled. Not knowing which book to select, you would have a hard time picking one up. Let's assume now that you decided to pick one up purely based on instincts. A second later, you start doubting the book's credibility. You then decide to go for another, and then another. Each one of these books has its own versions of answers, tips, and suggestions. Even if by some miracle you learn all of them, most of these would fail to work. The real problem lies in figuring out which one does.

The internet is exactly like that massive library, with almost no restriction on who posts what. This means you will come across hundreds of thousands of answers yet still not be able to figure out which one works. I don't know you personally, but I do know that you would never experiment on your baby. Our babies are our greatest treasures. There is no way we would experiment on them unless we have either heard about a certain method through someone we trust or read about it somewhere that is deemed as a credible and reliable source of information.

To save you from that hassle, I decided to dive deep into the world of myths, old wives' tales, and all of the things people have either said or posted online, and debunk each one of them to bring you to a logical conclusion. Whether you go for these or not is your choice altogether.

The main goal behind this exercise is to save you time and energy so that when the time comes, you know exactly what needs to be done to comfort your baby. Oh, and the neighbors who apparently know everything, you can politely let them know, "Hey, about that. It doesn't work!"

Honey, I Found This on the Internet

The internet is just one source. There are many other ways you may learn something new on how to keep your baby healthy, safe, and happy. You might encounter a friendly fellow shopper at your local baby store, and they may actually have something productive to say. You might tune into a TV show and you might just pick something up. It can be any source at any given time. However, do not fall for the obvious trap that most first-time parents do.

Do not carry out a certain action without due verification. One great way is to access websites that have credibility, such as the

American Academy of Pediatrics. Such sources are generally brimming with useful information and help you with great strategies to further ease the difficulty of the early parenthood phase.

There was once a couple who had a healthy baby boy. The baby was born without any signs of ailments or underlying conditions. One night, the child had a high-grade fever. Instead of calling a doctor or seeking medical attention, they decided to use a cold water bath. The baby was around seven months old at the time, so they were able to draw some water and let the baby sit in the cold water. While the baby's temperature dropped, something else happened that would leave the child scarred for life.

The sudden temperature change in the body caused the child's brain to cease normal function. According to the doctors, some of the nerves within the brain, which transmit signals from one end to the other, were no longer functioning. The child grew up to be intellectually impaired. He is 25 years old, yet he cannot speak, communicate, respond to his name, or even pay attention to anyone. The poor parents must always be home to ensure that their son does not step outside alone as he would have no memory of where he lives or how to get back.

All of this was caused because the parents had 'heard' of a way to quickly normalize high-grade fevers. Ever since I learned of this, I have been intentional about letting others know to truly verify their sources before proceeding to do something to ease a child's fever, or cater to any of their needs.

There are many such myths and so-called tips out there, circulating the internet and beyond. As parents, it is our desire and responsibility to do what is best for the child. By knowing what works and what doesn't, you can always be confident and be able to correct anyone who may think otherwise. With that said, let's dive into some of these myths and see what's what.

Newborns Can't See

I do not know who came up with that one, but what puzzles me, even more, is the fact that some parents actually believe such myths. Babies can see, which is why newborns keep looking around the room every now and then. This is the same reason why they respond by trying to grab their mother's breast because they can see that their source of nourishment is close. If you would like further evidence of this point, try and talk to your baby and see how they look right back at you before deciding to continue on exploring their surroundings.

Newborn Have Limited Sight

Okay, this one is actually true. Newborns can see everything up to a certain distance, generally three to five feet, after which everything is super blurry. Beyond this, newborns cannot see what or who may be on the other side of the room. Their world is quite literally tiny, which is why they seem to respond best when you are close.

In both of these cases, the thing to note is simple. Due to the fact that they can see, albeit limited, try not to shine bright lights directly into their eyes. This can hurt them and even cause sight issues. Keep direct light away and ensure their room has soft, warm lights. Use light diffusers to make the lights feel subtle and pleasing to the eyes.

Newborns Can't Hear

I'm sorry, but who is coming up with this stuff? People today say just about anything, without realizing the harsh results it could bring for the parents and the child. A baby gains a sense of hearing well before their actual birth. They can listen to pretty much everything that is going on outside, while still being inside their mother's womb.

This then brings us to a realization. When babies are a few months away from birth, avoid stepping into places with a lot of noises. Also, keep those noises down when the baby has come out and is in the crib or in the cozy arms of a parent. These noises can startle them, scare them, and might even make them wet themselves.

Babies Cannot Recall Anything Before Birth

Honestly, even I was skeptical of this one. How could a baby remember or recall anything while they were inside the womb? As it turns out, I was wrong.

Babies, since they can hear, have shown signs of remembering and recalling specific voices or melodies and can easily distinguish the ones they heard constantly while being inside the womb from ones that are unfamiliar.

Bravo, your child is already a genius! As astonishing as this is, it is also a bit of a warning for parents who may be expecting their baby soon.

I know couples tend to argue every now and then. However, during the last few months of pregnancy, try and avoid any kind of verbal altercations. Just remember, someone else other than you two can hear you scream and shout. Whether or not it could have any effect on the child's temperament is still being debated. Regardless, why take chances, right?

For parents who are preparing themselves to welcome their baby, pick out a nursery rhyme or a piece of music that is sweet and calm. Keep singing or playing it often. Once your baby comes, you can play that same music and the baby will instantly recognize it. If it is calm in nature, the baby will surely sleep easily.

Your Baby's First Smile Isn't Exactly a Smile

"Huh?"

That is exactly what I said when I came across this one. Apparently, there is a myth that a baby does not actually smile the first time. It is more of a reflexive action after passing gas.

As funny as this may sound, there is some truth in this. You see, newborns have no concept of what a smile is or why is it done in the first place. You may stare at your baby and smile every time, the baby simply reflects the action back to you without intent. That's just a reflex. It is only after the baby has grown up to be a few months old, or near the year mark, that they understand what a smile is.

The next time you see your newborn smile, don't suddenly jump to the conclusion that your baby wants to play. Give it a few seconds and try to find out if the baby may be passing gas instead of intentionally smiling. Don't keep them up by thinking they wish to play.

The Sudden Flailing and Movement Means the Baby Is Having a Seizure

No, no, no! It is stuff like this that often leaves parents worried beyond imagination. Parents, please do not fall for such nonsense. I am sure that by now you already know what this sudden flailing and movement indicate. Even if, for any reason, you are left scratching your head, let me reassure you it is nothing more than the baby feeling startled by some kind of sudden, unexpected, and loud sound.

I am not ruling out the possibility of a baby suffering from seizures, not at all. However, there is a significant difference between the two. If the baby flails immediately after a loud sound, there is absolutely nothing to worry about. It's just like you walking down a dark corridor and someone decides to jump right before you and yell, "Boo!"

In rare cases though, if there was no loud or unexpected sound that could have triggered this movement, it is probably best you consult a doctor right away. Never take chances but that does not mean that you will end up with the worst-case scenario. Calm yourself down and collect your thoughts, most of the time there is nothing to fear.

If your baby is sleeping, or about to fall asleep, and they flail a bit, it is okay. Just be there for the baby, and the baby should fall back to sleep almost immediately.

Don't Hold Your Baby Too Much, It Might Spoil Them

Holding a baby in your arms is a natural way to show affection towards the baby. There is absolutely no scientific evidence that suggests holding your baby a little too much would spoil them.

Feel free to hold your baby for as long as you like. Just be sure to put them to sleep when they start showing signs of tiredness. An agitated baby can often cry loud and for a while before going to sleep. Avoid that by picking up on the signs beforehand and the rest should be a piece of cake.

Swaddling Can Restrict Limb Growth

Swaddling is a technique that you are already familiar with by now. It is designed to comfort the baby and ensure the baby sleeps peacefully. Another advantage of swaddling is that a baby may not feel startled as easily as they feel that they are well protected.

Swaddling your baby does not restrict their growth and development of muscles or limbs at all. There is no scientific data to suggest that either. However, the American Academy of Pediatrics does recommend that you keep the hips section loose, to allow the hip some mobility, in case the child wants to move a bit. The hip section can face some complications if you wrap the baby up a bit too tightly. Always ensure that you leave the hip section a little loose as I described in the first chapter. The rest should just be fine.

Allergies Are More of a Genetic Thing for Babies

I have seen parents who try not to provide their newborns and children with specific fabrics, meals, or try and avoid cow's milk due to their own lactose intolerance. The fact is that your allergies or intolerance does not genetically pass on to your child. You may have an allergic reaction to nuts, but your children won't necessarily share that same allergy.

Babies are separate beings. Treating them based on your own experiences, good or bad, might have varying results. It is best to treat a baby just as a baby should be treated. You will find out about their potential allergies as they grow up.

You Can't Have Coffee When Breastfeeding

If you thought I forgot about you, don't worry. Breastfeeding is generally the option most opt for. Through this, the child gets all the nutrition needed to grow stronger and healthier. However, there are quite a lot of restrictions when you are breastfeeding a child.

To start, there are many medicines that you cannot consume when breastfeeding. This is due to the fact that some chemicals may enter the baby's digestive system through your milk. This can potentially have bad to worse consequences. But what about coffee? Can you have a cup of coffee to re-energize you during the morning, noon or night?

There is a myth that says you cannot. Following the same principle that the caffeine will find its way into the baby, this myth says coffee during breastfeeding is a bad idea. Here's some good news though: you can have up to five 5-ounce cups of coffee a day if you like.

While I wouldn't suggest you to go for such a high dose, you can certainly enjoy your coffee as you will need all the energy you can find to breastfeed the child multiple times a day. Now, thanks to some good old coffee, things will be a bit easier.

No Smoking or Drinking During Breastfeeding

Ouch! I know how hard it can get when you are told you cannot smoke or drink. Experts have unanimously declared both smoking and drinking extremely dangerous for the child who may be on breastfeeding. This means you will have to kiss your favorite packs of cigarettes, and those tempting bottles goodbye.

While there are thousands of other myths that you can come across the internet, here are a few more, specifically regarding the baby's sleep.

But Wait, There's More!

Hopefully, by now you are feeling a bit more educated and a little more confident regarding parenting your child. I am sure you may have actually come across a few of these myths before. In either case, it is your right to know what is best for your child. At the same time, through debunking these myths, you now have every idea of what is normal and what you should be worried about, in case something different happens.

Knowing these myths is only part of the learning curve, the actual intention is to enable you to act accordingly. By knowing all these myths about how a baby responds to sounds and how they see the world, you should feel a little more confident in the way you handle the affairs of the baby.

With that said, however, we will now look into some of the old wives' tales and some other suggestions which are always supposed to be avoided as these can either disturb the baby's sleeping habits or generally be harmful to the baby. It is a good idea to note these down so that you know exactly what to avoid that can cause your baby to have problems, negligible or otherwise.

Say No to Using Cold Water to Treat Baby's Fever

If you would recall, I mentioned a couple who faced one of the worst outcomes of following a so-called remedy blindly. The outcome saw the child permanently brain-damaged, and no science in existence can reverse the catastrophic impact it had on the child.

If your baby develops a fever, use lukewarm water to bathe your child. Be careful when you do so as deeper tubs can spell trouble. Alternatively, consult a specialist who can properly guide you to resolve the issue. Do not be tempted to carry out a certain action just because someone you know said so.

Always Opt for Dream Feed

For those who may have never heard of a dream feed, it is almost exactly as it sounds. This is done usually between 10 pm and midnight. This is the time when babies normally feel sleepy or are already asleep. Surprisingly, they still have this masterful ability to drink milk while they are asleep. The best part is, there is no reason to panic here either.

While many believe that this may lead to a baby choking on milk, the truth is quite the opposite. During these times, if you train yourself to feed the baby during their sleep, the baby will sleep longer and more peacefully.

This has to do with the fact that they will have a full belly for a longer duration of time. The longer the belly is full, the easier it is for the baby and even the parent to sleep. Practice dream feed and you can thank me later.

Give Some Time to Yourself and Your Partner

As odd as this would sound, the fact is that babies only need you until they fall asleep. If you follow the right methods and timing, your baby should sleep well, meaning that you have all the time for yourself.

A lot of people say they feel selfish for squeezing out time for themselves or their partners. There is no need to feel that way. Yes, the baby deserves all the love and care in the world, but so does your own body, mind, and soul. Let's not forget, we are human beings, we have needs and desires which we must fulfill every now and then. As a couple, your significant other may feel left out and that might strain relationships as well.

Find the right balance between your own life and the time you dedicate to the baby. The happier and more relaxed you are, the better you can care for your child.

White Noise Is Bad for Newborns?

Quite the contrary. White noise devices are selling like hotcakes these days. These have shown to work like a charm for parents who find it hard to put their kids to sleep.

If you remember from earlier how babies tend to recall sounds they may have heard while they were inside the womb, it is essentially the same thing happening here. When a baby is within the womb, they hear all kinds of sounds which we normally would not. This includes the beating heart of their mother, the blood rushing through her body, the breaths she draws in and out, and all of this is perfectly replicated by white noise devices.

Using sound machines does not harm your child's ability to hear in any way, shape or form. Therefore, consider this as an investment worth your money and time. The results are rather astonishing and fascinating, to say the least.

When turned on, these devices provide babies with a feeling of comfort and gives them a womb-like environment that has always shown to help babies go to sleep faster.

Besides, the white noise device is designed to act as an invisible sound shield that blocks off most of the noisy disturbances around the room including doorbells and other sudden or loud noises. Granted, they do not block them completely, but they do tend to bring the noise level down to a comfortable level (Lascurain, 2019). The conclusion is that your child can sleep more easily and you can carry on with your business as usual.

Keeping the Baby Awake Throughout the Day

I have often come across people saying that babies sleep more easily and longer at night by keeping them up during the day. Sorry, but it doesn't work that way.

If anything, you are only going to make your baby agitated and possibly even ill. Keeping them from falling asleep during the day, instead of allowing naps will only add anxiety and excessive tiredness to the baby. If you have been following closely, you would already know a tired baby will cry their heart out until they are put to sleep.

Do not keep your babies up. If anything, try and stick to a schedule where nap times are for the day and sleep time is for the night. Babies actually get used to fixed schedules easily and will tend to follow those accordingly. Furthermore, there is no evidence to suggest that the baby will sleep longer even after being up throughout the day.

Now, you can bury all of these scary myths, wives' tales, and claims which you may come across at some point in time, and do so with confidence. Remember, you are the best person for the job because you are the parent of the baby. It is only natural that you would only wish to do what is best for your child. By knowing some of these most commonly mentioned myths and remedies, you will know which ones actually work and how you can use them to make things better for yourself and for your baby. Always double-check the source. When in doubt, speak to an expert for a second opinion before you go on trying anything that may not sound right because it probably isn't.

Chapter 4:
Lullabies - Not the Only Way

Sometimes you have done everything by the book. You have played with the baby, kept them as active as possible after their naps. You have fed the baby with milk or formula, and the baby has also burped. Despite all that, the baby is unable to sleep.

"Not to worry, I will use the white noise device."

Well, not a bad call, to be honest, but let us assume for a second that you do not have one of those or that you are not exactly fond of using technology near a baby, what do you do then? A lullaby, of course.

Lullabies have been around for centuries, and maybe even more. Lullabies are essentially songs you sing which are deliberately soft in nature and sung in a melodious voice with minimal intensity. These have been suggested, recommended, and advised by hundreds of thousands of parents from generation to generation. The fact is, it does work!

Science has backed the significance and effectiveness of singing a lullaby to a baby. Experts from around the globe concede that singing lullabies to a baby provides them with relief, comfort, and promotes sleep. Before you know it, your child will be fast asleep in your arms.

Anyone can sing a lullaby, you do not necessarily have to be a singer or a musician in order to do this. As long as you can keep your vocal intensity down and use a soft tone, you are good to go.

Lullabies are one of the most effective ways to put your baby to sleep at night. This is where I am expecting that you read my last sentence properly. Lullabies are just one of many other ways to put your child to sleep. Previously within this book, we have discovered a few already, but now we will further dive into the details and see how each one of them works.

You do not necessarily need to know the science behind these methods as long as they work for you. However, I highly encourage that you at least know some basics before you proceed. This way, you will know what goes on and how you can make the most of the situation.

In this chapter, we will walk through:

- How lullabies work

- How to sing a lullaby

- Other forms and devices which do almost the same thing

Gear up, grab your pen and your paper and take notes when possible. First stop, lullaby town!

Rock-A-Bye Baby

Lullabies are generally sung by mothers to their babies. This does not mean that fathers cannot try and have a go at it. If you are a father, and you wish to sing a lullaby to your child, go for it. However, I would like to point out that mothers are more likely to gain success due to the fact that their naturally soft tone of voice is probably more pleasing to the baby, and additionally because the baby is used to hearing their mother's voice since a few months before birth.

Lullabies are effective because of three main reasons.

1. They are extremely effective in helping to regulate the baby's emotions.

2. These have shown a tendency to further enhance the bond between a child and their parent.

3. They are used to help establish a schedule or routine.

Already, the lullaby is proving to be a little more effective than we thought, right? Besides, the more we know the better. Well, we have a lot more to discover, so let's get to the point here.

How Lullabies Regulate Emotions

It is a world-known fact that music is not limited by age. Music, regardless of its kind, is heard, accepted, felt, and liked by every age group, whether a baby or an adult. Music is known to help regulate our emotions, and the same works for children as well.

Whenever your child is unable to sleep, it is only natural that you would try to do something to change that situation by controlling their emotions somehow. With a bit of practice, you can turn their fear or anger into something a little less intimidating.

With babies, who are under six months of age, finding out what they may be feeling is a bit tricky. If you do not know what they may be feeling, you may not be able to control the situation. However, with the help of a good lullaby, or preferably the one you sang a few months before your child's grand debut, you can stimulate some positive emotions through neural connections. Confused? Let me put it in another way.

Imagine a heartbroken guy, who just came out of a bad break-up. What kind of music do you think this person would prefer listening to? Quite obviously, it would most definitely be some kind of a sad score. The reason behind this is that they try and control their emotional response by relating to the music which makes them feel a little bit better. The music was able to change their state of mind and promote positive emotions for the person.

In quite the same fashion, a lullaby can distract the child's mind and make them feel better, relaxed, and comfortable. Soon enough, they will be so comfortable that they yawn and stretch before finally retiring to bed, or at least sleeping in your arms.

How Lullabies Create Better Bonds

Have you ever heard of a field of study called neurosciences? If not, it is the study of the nervous system within our bodies. Since our nerves are directly responsible for carrying a signal from one part of the body to another, whatever we feel, relate to, understand, and perceive theoretically falls under this field. When it comes to forming bonds, strengthening them, or losing them, it is also a part of neuroscience.

The reason I brought this up is that our bodies contain a specific hormone called oxytocin. This hormone is released by the body when we sing. This song-induced, special type of hormone is what causes us to feel the love around us, and this hormone is also referred to as the cuddle hormone. In short, it makes you feel like cupid struck you once again. This special type of hormone is what makes our bonds a bit deeper with the child.

Now, there is a little catch to this entire hormone and its production within our body. If you were to just sing the lullaby half-heartedly, this hormone is less likely to be produced by the body.

"Oh, you sly devil!"

Yes. This means you actually have to sing a lullaby as if you mean it, to ensure this hormone comes out and allows you to bond even better with your child. The magic here is the fact that the child feels the same way as well. This means this love isn't just a one-way affair. Your child will feel more secure, more loved, and will love you back equally. The results are, of course, a baby who falls asleep ever so peacefully.

How It Helps Create a Routine

Lullabies are one effective way to establish a set schedule for your baby's sleep pattern. If you pay a visit to an expert, you will come across advice that stresses the importance of establishing some kind of schedule for both the parents and the kids.

A baby is growing up, and this is the time when you can teach the baby to adapt to changes easily. By repeating the same actions at a specific time at night, every night, the baby will soon grow used to them and will stop resisting or paying attention to anything else but your voice. Up to this point, a child's mind is receiving signals that are indicating that their sleep time is upon them. The sooner they can start picking that up, the easier it will be for them to accept those signals and fall asleep.

Besides, lullabies have some other great benefits which can help your baby to grow more than just a sleeping habit. Lullabies can:

- Stimulate language easily

- Stimulate cognitive development

- Improves the memory and it helps increase the attention span

- Decreases stress and anxiety

Lullabies are a great way to not only put your baby to bed, but also to bond with them on a whole new level. Do not shy away from singing just because you don't consider yourself a singer. Do it for the child, and trust me you will feel so much better when you get to feel that love and see your baby slowly close those adorable eyes and fall asleep.

Now comes the part where I tell you some other things you can do to either add to the lullaby and make it more effective, or to do separately, in case the lullaby does not work for you.

So There's More Than Just Lullabies?

There are many ways through which you can put your baby to sleep. Singing a lullaby was only one method. As it turns out, you already know of another one. We came across it not too long ago. If you recalled it, bravo! If you couldn't, try and note it down as it greatly helps you to remember. I am indeed talking about the white noise device.

The white noise device has actually just surfaced in recent times. A few years ago, no one even knew they existed. They are small, cheap, and mighty effective. The problem is that not everyone is comfortable with the idea of having an electronic device near their newborn child. I do not know how you feel about it, therefore, I leave it up to you to decide.

We have already gone through the science behind the white noise and how it makes the baby feel more comfortable mimicking how the baby would have felt back before birth. Yes, this device is good for two reasons, eliminating noise and promoting sleep, but there are a few things you, as parents, should know.

Firstly, the white noise device is not necessarily suitable for all children. While the probability is high that they will enjoy it, there are always chances that your child may not like having this device around. If you do not see improvement in your child's sleeping habits, and if they do not fall asleep within five minutes, it is time to let go of the device.

Note: To fully be sure, try the device at least for three nights before coming to a conclusion.

Secondly, there is the noise that it makes. Yes, it is soothing for the child, it makes them feel like they are back in the womb, of sorts, but it is a noise in its own right. Noises can at times be too loud. Remember when I said that white noise does not harm a child? I meant it. It is not the white noise that can harm or disturb a child, but crossing a certain intensity would certainly agitate the child and the child may start crying, indicating that they want this noise to end.

If you are thinking of going for one of these devices, aim for the finest range. They are more likely to work and provide results. If white noise is not your thing, there is another way you can promote sleep, without actually buying separate toys or devices.

Using Lights the Right Way

Light plays an important part in a child's sleep routine which, surprisingly, many first-time parents and even experienced parents tend to overlook or even ignore. The amount and intensity of light within a room can greatly help you keep your baby active or it can invoke sleepiness in a child. Using it correctly can greatly bring you a bit of ease in the entire parenting process.

When I say lights, I mean both the natural and the artificial light. During the day, the daylight can allow a baby to feel more energized and to be more active, keeping the baby from sleeping. Since the intensity of the light is bright and high, it can be hard for a baby to sleep in such conditions. Open the windows or the blinds to let the bright daylight in when it is time for junior to wake up and do their usual activities, such as showing signs of excitement, feeding and giggling. Having the bright lights around will establish a habit where the baby would automatically know that the brightness indicates it is time to play.

When you see signs of tiredness, close the blinds to change the ambiance to a cozy, more relaxing one. The new light conditions will automatically allow your child to feel more comfortable, and the rest should be plain and easy.

Light tends to have a natural effect on human bodies, and it is equally felt by both children and adults. The newborns, up until the age of six months, tend to show a little more responsiveness to light than others. Consider the light as a source that pushes the baby's biological 'go' button (Pantley, 2017).

On the other hand, the absence of light also plays an important part. The darkness is what causes our brains to release melatonin, a hormone that is needed for us to sleep. By ensuring that the baby gets to play in well-lit conditions during the day and experiencing the darker nights, the baby will soon adapt to the settings and ease into the concept of sleeping well during nights.

Yes, it does take time as nothing about parenting is achievable overnight. It is this constant strive, this seemingly endless struggle that makes us parents. This is exactly why when we see our baby fall asleep, we forget about all the efforts, the aching back, the twisted ankle, and the headaches, we just savor the moment as we witness our little angel snoring away.

Now that you know the science behind it, it is time to make a to-do list for yourself. In this list, we will note down some important things we need to consistently do on a daily basis until the baby gets accustomed to these new changes.

Daytime

- Let the daytime be bright for the child.

- Allow plenty of sunlight to pour in your house.

- Take your baby outside for a bit of a stroll, as it helps you feel better as well.

- For daytime naps, let them nap in well-lit conditions. This ensures babies do not sleep more than usual and wake up in an hour or two at most.

- Plan most of the activities for the baby within the daytime.

Night

- If you haven't already done so, install dimmers on your lights and use these.

- Lower the lights at least two hours prior to the baby's sleep time (helps to set the mood).

- You can use a night-light in the baby's room, but ensure it is small and preferably one that remains cool, in case the baby touches it.

- If your baby wakes up during the night time, do not turn the lights on or carry the baby out into a well-lit area. This can trigger the baby's mind that it is time to get up.

- Keep all other light sources off or away to ensure a peaceful ambiance.

Follow these tips for a few days and your baby should soon grasp the concept of day and night. That will also allow sleep to take over its natural order. As long as there are no other distractions, the baby should sleep just fine, giving you a much-needed break during the day and good sleep during the night.

I will never promise that you can catch all your eight hours a day in one go. It is next to impossible as the baby continues to wake up and cry intermittently. It is something we have to learn to live with until the child finally hits the age of two to three years old. This is when the child will follow a more consistent routine and you should no longer have to worry about sticking to a strict schedule, changing diapers, and soon enjoy those captivating moments without a worry in sight.

Babies generally take a while before they are able to adapt to changes. For having a good sleeping pattern, including longer sleep during the night time, do not expect these changes to arrive as you would like before your baby turns four months old. It is usually after this age that the baby will respond accordingly and sleep for longer hours without waking up during the night. Until that happens, the above techniques can certainly help you put the baby to sleep and catch some shut-eye yourself.

Four months may sound like a long time, but trust me, it will pass and soon you will be looking back at this very moment, recalling just how quickly the time went by. It is a process we all go through so that we can one day say, "I've been there."

Time to change gears and head into the world of baby monitors, those neat little devices which everyone so dearly loves. The next chapter will look into how they work, how to respond to these, what to avoid, and so on. We will also be looking at how using baby monitors can get you the time you need for yourself and the things you can catch up with while your baby is busy dreaming.

Chapter 5:
The Benefits of a Baby Monitor

Just like everyone knows what Facebook or YouTube is, baby monitors also have significant popularity with the masses. This fame is not just limited to the United States, it is equally popular in almost every other major country on earth. It does not take long to see why these are as popular as they have become.

Baby monitors function just as they sound; they monitor the baby's activity. The yesteryear's models were only focusing on sounds. Their sensitive microphones would pick up even the slightest sounds and transmit it across the room to the receiver. With technology advancing faster than we can keep pace with, there are newer models out in the market which offer all sorts of amazing features.

Today, you can buy a baby monitor that will not only capture sounds but will also show you the baby through the onboard video camera installed. These are great, and they sound worth buying, but do you really need one at all?

In this chapter, as promised earlier, we will look into some important aspects of the baby monitor and how much of a necessity it is. We will also be looking across a few variants and hopefully, understand which ones are a better alternative for our situation. Finally, we will be looking at one surprising entry. I assure you, it will be well worth the wait.

A Guardian Technology or a Noisy Speaker?

Technology has always surprised us with many great inventions which ease our way of living, in one way or another.

Most of these technologies have come and gone while some have struck a chord and turned from a luxury to a necessity. Baby monitors are no exception to the latter part. These handy little devices came out quite some time ago and have managed to stick around ever since.

Yes, these fascinating little devices continue to grow in numbers because of the sheer peace of mind that they bring for worrying parents. By having a third ear of sorts, you get to do whatever it is that you are doing, knowing that when the baby is up, you will be duly notified.

These devices have come a long way and it should be of no surprise that with time, these devices have become more technologically advanced. With features like live video stream, more accurate microphones, two-way communication, and motion sensors, you are sure to get your money's worth.

Now, before you actually decide to go for one of these little devices, there is a bit of advice which you must take into consideration and understand. These devices are meant for monitoring purposes, however, there is no way on earth that these are a substitute or an alternative that you can rely on upon alone. Personal monitoring and supervision are always the best and the safest way to go about raising your child. Use these only when your baby is in a perfectly safe sleeping zone, and when you are at home yourself.

Under no circumstances should you leave your baby home without a parent to look after them. Monitors are limited in functionality and cannot perform things which may be necessary at that point in time. They are strictly to be used as a way to detect the activity of a baby during sleep and serve as a way for you to know if you are needed in their room.

Okay, I am done sounding all bossy and scary. Let us resume learning things that really matter, and that leads us to a question. Why do we use baby monitors in the first place?

The most obvious reason is the fact that we cannot always be around the baby. There are things we need to do, chores we have to tend to and people we need to talk to. It is just how life is. We cannot stop living life just so we can be with the baby at all times. This is a natural order of things. Therefore, we go for a piece of technology that acts as our distant set of ears while we cook, do the laundry, greet the guests, have dinner, or even get intimate with the spouse. It is impossible to be in two places at once, and that is why these baby monitors are a blessing in disguise.

They offer us a chance to resume life, or at least most of it, and have peace of mind that we will be notified immediately if the baby is up, by transmitting the noise and lighting up those little green, yellow and red blips.

Besides the most obvious reason, there are other uses of baby monitors as well. These have more to do with the medical condition of your child. If your child was born prematurely, meaning before the due date, or has a breathing problem, you might be referred by a doctor to use one of the more advanced versions of these monitors. This specific type of monitor keeps monitoring your baby's heart rate and breathing rate. The doctors generally advise you to install these in your home to detect any issues with the baby's health.

This part is a little scary, I admit, but it is something you may wish to note. Whether it is your baby or someone you know has a baby with a breathing problem, you can use this information to evaluate if you need these specialized baby monitors.

A doctor would recommend these if the baby:

- Has already shown a need for resuscitation (meaning that the baby may have been found not breathing or bluish in color)

- Has a prolonged pattern of pauses while breathing

- Has a slow heart rate

- Has some kind of breathing disorder that may very well affect the baby during sleep

- Has some type of rare medical condition which may require oxygen at all times

If any of these are observed, these baby monitors will certainly be helpful. I do hope that no parent ever has to witness these difficult circumstances. It is a living nightmare to watch your baby in such a state and be able to do nothing about it. The best course of action in such situations is to get in touch with a doctor as quickly as possible and let them know what the readings are on the monitor. The quicker you act, the merrier the chances of a speedy recovery in most cases.

To summarize, you either use baby monitors to know when your baby needs you while you are in another room or another part of the home, or you use these to monitor the health of the baby.

Nowadays, there are a whole bunch of baby monitors you can buy from your local stores which can go a step further and provide you with a little more satisfaction. It does make sense to invest money into these advanced versions as the older ones would pick up any noise and keep the parents rushing to and fro for no reason. So what other types of monitors are there, and are they worth the hefty price tags?

Audio Monitor

This is the most basic of the lot. A simple device that transmits audio from one end to the other. Some advanced versions allow you to have a two-way communication as well. In case you want your baby to know that you are coming and hopefully cause the baby to calm down a little until you arrive, these can be good.

The problem is that these versions pick up every noise, and sometimes not all noises are worth attending. As surprising as this may sound, it is also not recommended that you rush right away if you hear a baby crying a little. Give it a minute, it just might be that your baby was spooked during sleep. Your baby might just nod off again. If the crying gets louder, that is your cue to rush.

If you can find yourself a brand that offers refined audio quality and some kind of control on what kind of noise level it should ignore, go for it. It is definitely beneficial to have one.

Video Monitor

For a bit more money, you can opt for a baby video monitor. This one can either stream live video feed to the receiving device, your laptop, tablet, or even your phone. If I was to choose the type of monitor I wanted for my baby, I would definitely go for one of these.

By having the baby monitor stream a high-resolution video, I would certainly know what the noise was and whether the baby is up or just mumbling in their sleep.

Movement Monitor

These are new and a bit more advanced. Usually installed underneath your baby's comfortable bedding, these send off alarms to a receiving device if your baby has failed to move during a set period of time. I am sure you are expecting me to add further features, but I promise, that is all it can do.

Honestly, these are expensive and a complete waste of money. However, that is my personal opinion. If you still wish to go for one, by all means, do so.

A New Alternative

Remember I said there is a surprise entry? What if I told you that you can have a baby monitor for free? That is exactly what you, or anyone else for that matter, can get.

All you need is a smartphone, android, or iOS, browse to your app store and search for a baby monitor. There are hundreds of apps that offer exactly the same functionality of an audio or a video baby monitor, and most of them are free to use. This means that you do not have to buy a separate baby monitor at all. How does it work? Simple.

You use a device, suppose a table you rarely use, and leave it at a place near to your baby's sleeping area. You set up the stream (audio or video), set the minimum noise level you want, and that is it. It will stream that video to any connected device and set off an alarm if the noise limit is breached.

In some cases, you can set up text alerts or call alerts as well. This means that when the baby is up or makes significant noise for a cellular device to pick up, it will automatically send out a text or a pre-recorded call stating that the baby is up. Genius! However, their quality is not exactly the best, especially the video feeds. They seem choppy and they do have a nasty pixelated effect on most of these apps. But hey, it's free and it is still getting the job done.

Using any kind of baby monitor is okay, and dare I say even recommended. As long as you know you are within the house and that you are not using headphones to listen to music or do something that may block out the noise, it should actually be useful. Always remember that a baby monitor is essentially an alarm; its purpose is only to warn you and that is it. It will not save your baby's life or put the baby back to sleep in any way. Relying on these is okay, but relying on them alone is not at all advised nor recommended.

I Bought One, Now What?

Oh, so you got yourself a baby monitor? As eager as I would be to find out the make, model, and type you opted for, I will skip that and get straight to the point.

The baby monitor is up and running, your child has just finished having a healthy dose of milk, and you have just put your baby to bed. Now comes the part where your other aspects of life can be catered to. However, don't go rushing into a warm bath just yet. Think things through and use the time to do the necessary tasks first. I assure you, for the first few months, it gets really hard for us parents to manage time. There is just so much to be done in so little time.

The first order of the day is to set up a to-do list. Use post-it notes or sticky notes, or even the notes on your cell phone, and start prioritizing what you need to get done today or tomorrow. I personally would recommend that you set up a to-do list the night before and simply cross out the ones you complete. Your goal is not to complete the list, but to do the ones which are most important.

There are a few things you cannot do, such as go shopping or do your groceries, unless you either have your spouse stay home and watch the baby or you both decide to take the baby with you instead. In either case, the baby must not be left alone.

Household chores, such as doing the dishes, making dinner, cleaning the house, and so on, can be done one by one during the day time naps of the baby. Simply keep the receiving unit of the baby monitor with you and continue doing your work. It greatly helps if your partner is also involved as it can rapidly reduce the workload and get the job done quicker. Plus, it is also going to strengthen your bond.

While doing house chores, try not to make too much noise. Vacuum cleaners are okay to use but if you are near your baby's room, skip it for now until the baby is up. If you are watching the news or tuning in to your favorite TV show, be sure to turn the volume down a bit. This is to ensure that the baby monitor is still audible and that the baby doesn't get startled from any sudden noise that may pop up.

Self-care, such as workouts or personal hygiene can be taken care of while your baby is napping. Remember, you will only have a window of one to three hours at most before your baby is awake once again. Choose wisely what you wish to do and enjoy your time.

Moving on to night time, you have your dinner, do any last-minute chores, all of which can be done when the baby is up. This is where the baby monitor is not needed unless your baby is already asleep.

If your baby is up, having dinner while holding the baby can be dangerous. Investing in a baby carrycot would be advisable as you can simply put your baby in the cot and near you while you two have your dinner. A toy or two might keep them occupied while you eat. Once done, have one partner do the dishes while the other feeds the baby.

Now comes the time for bed. Set up your baby monitor, dim those lights, and eliminate all loud sources of sound and music before you finally put the baby to bed. Hopefully, by this time, you would have had a couple of hours to spare before you call it a night.

Use this time to be there for each other. Catch up on a new movie on your favorite streaming service or do some gaming, if that is your thing. Alternatively, you can use this time to engage in intimacy which you can fully enjoy because you know you have a third ear that is keeping track of your baby.

Baby monitors are certainly a good buy, but there is no point in buying one if you do not intend to use it properly and utilize the extra advantage you gain out of it. Use it well, use it wisely, and above all, use it safely.

In this chapter, we looked at what we could use to further ease our lives and ensure that our baby sleeps well and safely. In the coming chapter, we will be looking at things from the perspective of the baby, including what tools a baby can use to assist themselves.

Chapter 6:
The Tools for the Little Ones

This may have come to you as a bit of a surprise, but the fact is that babies also have certain tools that they can use for their own comfort. While there is a debate on whether or not these 'tools' are exactly necessary for children, it is absolutely your call regarding how you wish to view these.

Babies put on quite a show most of the time, and it all is very adorable, cute, and sweet. Then there are times where they put on a different kind of show, unexpected, unnerving, and annoying. These are bouts of crying out loudly, at times for no obvious reason at all, and handling such issues can leave even the most experienced parent in doldrums. Fortunately, though, there are a few things which can help us deal with such situations. These are things which we have seen and heard of but have never really taken into consideration.

There are a number of items that come to mind, but we are not here to start buying each one of them. Instead, we will be looking at the ones which specifically contribute to the general well-being and safety of the child. We will go through the list of these items which have shown promising results in aiding us to put the baby to sleep or keep them calm and happy when things seem to go a bit rough.

While we may buy them, rest assured that they are not yours at all. A baby, despite their age, knows how to demand something and they do so with authority. Parents can't really help but to fulfill these demands. Fortunately, most of these are safe and actually help us in a way. These can help keep your baby at ease when visiting a crowded place like a mall, or they can promote sleep so that the baby sleeps even in conditions other than the one they may be used to. Let's dive in and see what's what.

Note: This may seem like a buyer's guide, but hey, as long as it works, it is worth it.

Oh, I Want One!

This list, or any other list of baby essentials, is incomplete without a pacifier. It is one of the most iconic and soothing inventions that has kept millions of babies quiet, providing them with a comfort that only they can feel and has kept parents away from all that noise and drama.

I do not know who named these but whoever you were, bravo! These truly get the job done in most cases. Have a fussy baby? No problem. Give your child a pacifier and watch the magic happen before your own eyes. Within an instant, your baby would be sucking away at the pacifier and genuinely show happiness.

It is observed by Mayo Clinic, a renowned name in its own right, that babies are generally happy when they are sucking on something. Pacifiers offer them a soft, rubbery surface that is clean, hygienic, and safe, which they can nibble and suck on for hours at a stretch.

Pacifiers may seem to be all about calming your baby down and helping them to sleep, however, these have both pros and cons which you should take into consideration before you opt for one.

Pros:

- Pacifiers are known to calm most babies down.

- Pacifiers are great as a temporary distraction, which is why most babies will immediately go quiet when they start sucking on one. Imagine your baby just receiving their scheduled shots, tests, or blood tests. These will distract them and soothe their minds right away.

- Pacifiers have shown to be of great help to put your baby to sleep.

- For parents thinking of flying with a baby, a pacifier can help them fight the altitude discomfort.

- Pacifiers just might help to reduce the risk of Sudden Infant Death Syndrome (SIDS).

- These are disposable. This means, when the pacifier starts to look murky, is torn or if you want your baby to break the habit, simply discard them.

Cons:

- Using pacifiers at an early age (before four weeks) may interfere with the breastfeeding process.

- There is a chance that your baby may become dependent on these pacifiers. This generally happens if you allow babies to use pacifiers every now and then.

- Pacifiers may increase the risk of developing middle ear infections.

- Using pacifiers over prolonged periods of time can often lead to dental issues. It is okay to use pacifiers during the first few years, but anything after that may cause permanent dental issues like misaligned teeth.

All of this then is your call. Whether you choose to go for a pacifier or not is debatable. There is no harm in going for one, as long as you can follow some guidelines. These guidelines are designed to ensure the safety of your child.

- Do not introduce a pacifier before breast-feeding is well adapted. The American Academy of Pediatrics highly recommends that you wait until your baby is three to four weeks old before introducing a pacifier.

- Pacifier is not your go-to solution. Do not use these as your first line of defense. Try and rock your baby or change their position first to see if that calms them down. Only use pacifiers between feeding sessions.

- If your baby does not like the pacifier, it is best not to force it. If your baby is asleep and the pacifier falls down, do not put it back in their mouth.

- Choose wisely the type of pacifier you go for. It is recommended that you choose one-piece silicone, the dishwasher-safe type. The double piece may pose choking hazards.

- Always clean the pacifier before use. It is a good practice to clean the pacifier immediately after use and clean it once again before giving it to the baby.

- Never apply any sweet substance on top of the pacifier.

- Replace these as often as you can and choose the one that best suits your baby's age.

When your baby is around two years, it is time to pull the plug. First, try and let the baby stop using pacifiers on their own. If you see such behavior, encourage them by using kind words. If not, you can try and hide them or simply throw them away. Prolonged use would outweigh the benefits and that is not a situation we would like our babies to be in.

Apart from pacifiers, which evidently makes the baby feel at ease, there are other things to consider as well. One important thing to include here is the baby's wardrobe.

Yes, babies are quite picky when it comes to the kind of clothes they wear. They may not say much about the color, but make no mistake, they will let you know if the clothes they are wearing are comfortable or not.

I have seen parents who go for unbranded clothes that clearly do not reflect quality and safety. Later on, they complain that the fabric made their child itch or develop rashes followed by agonizing cries. Always ensure that you settle for the finest quality which is known to provide comfort and are free of any allergenic material.

For the wardrobe, you will need:

- Onesies (the ones which fold at the shoulder and snap at the crotch side)
- Shirts
- Pants
- One-piece pajamas
- Rompers
- Sweaters/Jackets
- Socks
- Hats
- Mittens (be sure to pick up the no-scratch range)
- Wearable blankets (for winters)
- Stroller blankets

These are just some of the most commonly used items you can come across. Ensure good quality and your baby should be experiencing comfort all round.

Apart from your baby's wardrobe solution, next comes toys. Before anyone else tells you that you need to buy a specialized series of toys in order to begin early learning, let me be honest with you. Babies do not learn anything such as alphabets, names of animals, and such until they reach at least 12 months of age. Spending a significant amount of money on these so-called early educational toys is simply a waste. At this point, all your baby needs is food and comfort, and that's it.

Between the ages of zero to six months, babies quite literally try and suck or bite on anything they can get their hands on. Avoid any toys which are not soft in nature, have parts that can come off easily, or have electronic components within them. Stick with perhaps the most demanded ones out there, both safe and chewable toys.

Babies just love chewable toys. One of the finest I remember is the chewable gel keys. They are made out of a gel-like substance which makes the toy feel cold to touch. Babies of three months and above love chewing on these and the best part is that they are free of any harmful chemicals. By chewing, babies get a soothing sensation and that also takes away any itch they may have within their gums.

Chewable toys are great, but they are mostly meant for children who are at least three months old. These are a great addition to the toolbox besides a pacifier and some comfortable clothes. They can keep the kids distracted and allow them to have a bit of fun while they are at it.

Next stop, we have the rocking chair, or perhaps a glider. The latter only sounds like something an adult would use to fly around cities and higher grounds, but in reality, these are far safer and easier to use.

These essentially allow babies to be rocked back and forth, providing the baby with a sense of calmness, peace and promotes sleep unlike any of the above-mentioned items. Personally, I would go for these over toys any given day. They help greatly, they are easy to clean, and in quite a lot of cases, very easy to carry as well. Whether you are visiting a friend, going out for a spot to picnic, or just trying to put your child to sleep, these work their magic instantly.

Here is yet another fine item on the list. If you live in a region where mosquitos and flies are a constant problem, I would highly recommend you get yourself a decent crib netting. These are designed to have enough space inside while having a fine netting to protect the baby from flies and mosquitos. This would allow your baby to sleep easily and leave you worry-free.

Finally, I understand how hard it can be to breastfeed babies in places other than home. It is a must that you get yourself a few bottles and nipples, along with other things like brushes and sterilizers. If you are breastfeeding, a breast pump would do nicely. You can bottle up your breast milk and feed it to the baby without drawing attention and feeling awkward. Alternatively, if you are not breastfeeding, you can whip up a batch of formula and go on feeding your child easily wherever you go.

It is essential that these bottles are safe, easily cleaned, and secure in nature. Always opt for bottles by recognized brands and manufacturers as lower quality items may cause issues and lead to complications for the baby.

I Gotta Get One Of These, Too!

Below are some other suggestions which may prove to be helpful to you. You can find most of these quite easily in all local baby stores and outlets.

- Cradle or bassinet

- Cool mist humidifier, as warm mist can sometimes breed bacteria

- Infant car seats

- Stroller

- Baby swing

- High chair for the baby

- Bibs

- Burp cloth

- Baby first aid kit and thermometer

- Diaper bag

- Diaper cream

- Baby bathtub

As always, buying some or all of these are a matter of choice and preference. It is not mandatory that you buy everything on the list. Aim only for items that genuinely help you and the baby in some way. Anything that is more of luxury is simply going to go obsolete in a year or so once the baby outgrows the need for such an item.

That would be pretty much everything to cover for this chapter. In our final chapter, we will quickly go through one aspect of the baby's routine that I mentioned earlier. I wanted to prioritize the important parts first so that the last chapter makes more sense.

Chapter 7:
The Importance Of Naps

Now that we know everything about what a baby needs, how a baby communicates, how to set a schedule and all of the essentials that we and the baby can use to have a good night's sleep, it is time to look at naps.

If you thought that naps are more of an adult thing, you were wrong. Babies love naps far more than we do. In fact, on average a baby sleeps every two hours. We cannot even think of doing something like that because that would get us fired from work, cause health issues, and make us look like lost causes. Things work a little differently when it comes to babies.

In this relatively smaller chapter, we will go through a few things which every parent should know about naps. It will reinforce the concepts and importance of naps for both parents and kids. Hey, if your child gets a nap, you get some rest too. By the time your child wakes up, you would also feel a lot better and energized.

It's Nappy Time

Our little bundle of joy is born to amaze us. From those subtle movements to their little snores, everything about the child is worth capturing on video to relive that feeling over and over again. Yes, throughout the book, we aimed to learn what it takes for parents, first-timers, or even the experienced ones, to put the baby to sleep and to keep them healthy and safe. Mostly, we focused on sleep, but finally, after knowing every tool in the box, you are now ready to learn the importance of naps.

It is only natural that babies nap a lot. It is just how babies develop their physical and mental abilities. Naps serve as their much-needed downtime. Since the child is just a few weeks or months old, the baby can easily get tired. Naps are a natural way to ensure that babies do not grow overtired.

By now, you already know what happens should a baby remain up for a longer period of time. The baby will get irritated, fussy and that spells trouble to the already exhausted parents. Failure to put a baby down for a nap can result in a harder time at night trying to put the baby to sleep.

Besides, parents need their downtime as well. Yes, we are supposed to rest six to eight hours a day, but adding a baby to the picture makes that seem like a distant dream. The only way to recover the lost sleep time is by taking a nap or at least a breather yourself. This is only possible if you are able to put your baby down for a good nap that extends from one to three hours at most. Anything more than that could only cause you additional issues during nighttime.

Your baby's daytime naps also allow you to carry out general household chores, in case you do not wish to delay those. Remember the to-do list we made earlier on? You can continue striking a few of those items off the list and may still be able to catch a quick nap.

Be sure that you do not include any activities that may produce a lot of noise as these can instantly startle the baby and wake them up. It is also recommended that you do not leave the baby alone in the house as the baby can wake out of the nap for any given reason.

Signs That Matter

There are ways to tell if your baby is getting enough sleep, including naps. Keep an eye out for signs such as:

- The baby is acting sleepy during the day

- The baby is cranky in the late afternoon

- The baby is giving you a hard time getting out of bed in the morning

- The baby is being inattentive, hyperactive or impatient

If you see any of these signs, it is probably because the baby is not able to get enough sleep. Naps can certainly ease the situation and bring the child back on a more scheduled sleep pattern.

For infants, if you see them rubbing their eyes or getting cranky, rock them a bit or use the rocking chair. Once the baby is feeling sleepy, but not yet asleep, put them to bed. Once you do this a few times, the baby will learn how to sleep on their own, and this will greatly help you with both nap times and nighttime sleep.

Not everything about parenting needs to be challenging, if you know what needs to be done and when, you can actually save yourself quite a lot of hassle.

Well then, it is now time for me to say, "Congratulations!" because you have shown a will to learn everything that has to do with putting babies to sleep and catching some rest yourself. I do not know who you are, where you may be on this green and blue planet of ours, but wherever you are, I want you to know this: you have all the willpower and determination that it takes to be a great parent.

We have gone through the ups and downs, discovered new techniques, debunked some classical myths, and even picked up a few words babies use to communicate. You made a few entries in your notebook, created a to-do list, and probably even scribbled some items to buy for your baby. I see no reason why you would fall into any trouble from here on out.

Parenting is tough, there is no denying that, but it is people like you who would go the extra mile to do what is right for your child that make and define the perfect parent. I honestly hope that you were able to gain a deeper understanding of our subject at hand. I would love to know how your journey goes from this point forward. I wish you only the best, and I hope you enjoy parenthood as much as possible. Savor every moment with your family, and always remember to be there for each other.

Conclusion

Wow! What began as a simple question soon turned into a complete book. Putting babies to bed, how hard can that be? As it turns out, not as easy as you might think.

To begin with, there are countless elements at play that influence your baby's mind. There are distractions, noises, the clothes they wear, the temperature around them, the list just keeps on going. Get any of these wrong and you are back to square one, with the addition of a crying baby, of course.

Parenting is seen as the toughest full-time job on the planet, and believe me when I say this: that is the understatement of the millennium. Parenting comes with both joys and an endless struggle. What seemingly is one of the easiest jobs turns into a full-blown nightmare if you have no clue what needs to be done. Luckily, you searched for an answer, and hopefully, you just found it.

Babies are super cute, adorable and they have the purest form of expressing their love, demands, and needs. They come into our world and apparently it feels like they are here to sleep it off. Newborns sleep almost all day, albeit in episodes. It is next to impossible to keep track of their sleeping behavior, and that is where most parents start worrying.

You never know when your child might wake up and demand to be fed. It could be from 1 am to 3 am, or it could be just an hour before your work begins. One thing is certain, babies need their sleep, and it is our job as parents to ensure that they get exactly that.

By observing how they sleep, when they sleep and for how long they sleep, we can soon start working out a schedule. This schedule will help us out once the baby grows a bit older. Later, we can introduce some more elements such as light conditions, electronic devices such as the white noise sleeping aid device, and others to promote longer sleeping hours.

Of course, not all is about the baby either. Parents are also human beings, and they need their rest as well. In order to keep pace with the baby and the piling workload, they too, need to ensure that babies sleep longer so that they can rest as well. It takes more than a single person to make things work. Dear mommy can take care of a few aspects while daddy dear can ensure that other tasks are taken care of.

Parents often seek out help and advice from other people, and worryingly, they use these tactics to experiment on their babies. That is a big no. Never try something you aren't sure of or have not researched yourself. Only stick to methods and techniques which are backed up by some credible sources or research. Simple errors and misunderstandings can often lead to dire circumstances, and that is a situation no parent would like to be in.

I am sure by now you are already familiar with some of these, and I sincerely hope that you would avoid such dangerous myths and old wives' tales at all costs. If you really need assistance, first observe what is wrong. It is very much possible that a quick visit to the baby store might just be the thing you need to do. Perhaps a toy or a pacifier to divert your baby's attention, or a rocking chair to put them to sleep easily. Whatever it may be, observe first, then approach an expert and discuss your concerns.

Finally, the arrival of a baby does not mean you go on spending a fortune on toys and needless items. Stick to the ones which are needed, safe, and recommended by experts. Pick out the ones that genuinely help you and the child in some way. Things like teether toys, crib nettings, and baby monitors are perhaps a good buy. Think things through and act accordingly.

You have every reason to be excited and be afraid at the same time. Parenthood is not everyone's cup of tea, and I assure you, you are not alone if you feel this way. The greatest fear a parent has is the fear of failure. With the dedication you have shown to go through all this information, I can honestly say that you have everything within you to make a great parent. With love, and a bit of willpower, you will pull through and before you know it, you will l be teaching others how to be great parents such as yourselves.

References

Assessments For Newborn Babies. (n.d.). Retrieved from
    https://www.stanfordchildrens.org/en/topic/default?id
    =assessments-for-newborn-babies-90-P02336

Baby Crying Sounds - What Do Different Cries Mean? (2018,
    August 17). Retrieved from
    https://www.petitjourney.com.au/understand-the-
    different-cries-of-your-baby/

Baby Monitors and Sensors. (2019, February). Retrieved from
    https://www.pregnancybirthbaby.org.au/baby-
    monitors-and-sensors

Ding, K. (n.d.). Expert sleep strategies for babies. Retrieved
    from https://www.babycenter.com/0_expert-sleep-
    strategies-for-babies_1445907.bc#articlesection1

How Baby Sleep Cycles Differ From Adult Sleep Cycles. (n.d.).
    Retrieved from
    https://www.sleepfoundation.org/articles/how-your-
    babys-sleep-cycle-differs-your-own

Pacifier do's and don'ts. (2017, July 22). Retrieved from
    https://www.mayoclinic.org/healthy-lifestyle/infant-
    and-toddler-health/in-depth/pacifiers/art-20048140

Pantley, E. (2017). The no-cry sleep solution for newborns.
    New York: McGraw-Hill Education.

Sparrow, J. (n.d.). Debunking Baby Myths. Retrieved from
    https://www.scholastic.com/parents/family-life/social-
    emotional-learning/development-
    milestones/debunking-baby-myths.html

Swaddling: Is it Safe? (2020, April 4). Retrieved from
     https://www.healthychildren.org/English/ages-
     stages/baby/diapers-clothing/Pages/Swaddling-Is-it-
     Safe.aspx

Tantum, J. (2019, April 11). Sleep expert shares top baby sleep
     myths. Retrieved from
     https://www.shepherdsfriendly.co.uk/your-resource-
     centre/baby-sleep-myths

The 6 Best Ways to Make Your Baby Tired (and 3 Things NOT
     to Do). (2019, March 15). Retrieved from
     https://health.clevelandclinic.org/the-6-best-ways-to-
     make-your-baby-tired-and-3-things-not-to-do/

www.ingramcontent.com/pod-product-compliance
Lightning Source LLC
Chambersburg PA
CBHW051221250726

48655CB00006B/2537